Eating awareness journal for emotional eaters

A Food Crazy Mind Journal
By Davina Chessid

Disclaimer: The information in this book is not intended as a substitute for the advice of trained medical or mental health professionals. The reader should consult his/her physician, therapist or counselor in matters relating to physical or mental health and particularly with respect to any symptoms that may require diagnosis or medical attention. In the event you use any of the information in this book, the author and the publisher assume no responsibility for your actions.

All rights reserved. No part of this publication may be reproduced, distributed, or transmitted in any form or by any means, including photocopying, recording, or other electronic or mechanical methods, without the prior written permission of the author and publisher, except in the case of brief quotations embodied in reviews and certain other non-commercial uses permitted by copyright law.

© 2016 Davina Chessid
www.foodcrazymind.com

CONTENTS

INTRODUCTION 1
IN THIS JOURNAL 3
HOW TO USE THIS JOURNAL 5
SPECIAL REPORT 7
    5 WAYS JOURNALING CAN STOP A BINGE 7
    DISTRACTION 9
    AWARENESS 11
    INSIGHT 13
    ACCOUNTABILITY 15
    SELF-CARE 17
MOTIVATIONS 19
EATING AWARENESS 29
    WEEK ONE 31
        Week One INSIGHTS 46
    WEEK TWO 51
        Week Two INSIGHTS 66
    WEEK THREE 71
        Week Three INSIGHTS 86
    WEEK FOUR 91
        Week Four INSIGHTS 106
JOURNAL PAGES 111

INTRODUCTION

I started journaling because I was out of control. I needed information about what I was thinking and doing... and about how I could make healthier choices.

In my journal, I wrote about my craziest moments with food. (Many of those entries made their way into the best-selling book, *Food Crazy Mind*.) The process of writing brought clarity and calmness to my mind and my eating.

I've heard it said that the five most frightening words in the English language are "it will change your life." If you've never really looked at what you're eating, keeping a food journal can be eye-opening!

According to doctors, nutritionists and diet gurus, keeping track of what we eat is key to creating a healthy relationship with food. It's necessary to understand our behavior if we want to make different choices and manage ourselves more effectively.

This journal is focused on creating awareness for those of us who struggle with emotional eating.

You'll be prompted to record what you eat and drink as well as your emotional state, so you can develop a greater understanding of the connections.

The awareness that comes with focusing your attention on your internal life and how it affects your eating is instrumental in making the change to a healthier, happier relationship with food.

Journaling helps, not just those of us who want to lose weight but those of any size who want to improve our habits around food.

Keeping track provides accountability, gives us information about what and how much we're eating (which isn't always what we think) and inspires us to pay attention.

If you struggle with emotional eating, binge eating or compulsive eating, if you're out-of-control when it comes to food, if you know what to do but you're not doing it... a journal can help you better understand yourself and what lies beneath your choices, so you can move towards different behaviors and different outcomes.

Use this journal yourself or bring it to your nutritionist, doctor, therapist or coach. It will help you on any eating plan.

Keep in mind that for most of us, change doesn't happen immediately, it's a process. Practice self-compassion and begin with a commitment to consciously learn about yourself. Make awareness, not perfection, your focus.

You **can** take control of your out-of-control eating.

IN THIS JOURNAL

- *Special Report: 5 Ways Journaling Can Stop a Binge,* including journaling prompts to help you deepen your understanding of your relationship with food. Journaling can help you avoid future binges and may even stop a binge in its tracks.

- Space to record your motivations: understanding your 'why' will keep you focused. Return to this section for inspiration.

- Four weeks of daily tracking your food and emotions.

- Space to track how you feel before, during and after you eat – with additional journal pages for each day to describe your emotions in greater detail.

- Weekly tracking of your insights and the connections between how you feel and what you eat.

- Space to record your ideas for the following week.

- A list of emotional words to help you articulate your feelings.

- At the back of this book you'll find additional blank, lined journal pages for further writing.

You're in great shape for the shape you're in.

-Dr. Seuss

HOW TO USE THIS JOURNAL

- Read the *Special Report: 5 Ways Journaling Can Stop a Binge.*
    - To respond to the prompts, you can use the journaling pages at the back of this book (beginning on page 115).
    - It's a great idea to use the journaling prompts as such, but even holding the questions in your thoughts as you move through the process of tracking your food and feelings, can be very helpful.
- Fill in the motivation pages and create your top 5 motivations for the next four weeks. You can return to this section for motivation.
- Use the Daily Tracking Chart and the Journaling Page opposite the chart to record what you eat and describe your emotions.
    - If possible, don't wait until the end of the day to write down what you consume and how you're feeling.
    - In the Daily Tracking Chart, use the column "How I Feel" to record - *in just a few words or less* - your general emotional state before, during and after you eat.
    - Use the Journaling Page (opposite the chart) to go into greater detail about your emotions

- by expanding on what you've written in the "How I Feel" column.
- Use the **Words of Emotion** list (page 34) to get you thinking about words that might accurately describe how you feel.
- At the end of each week, record your insights, as well as any patterns or themes you notice and any ideas you have for the following week.
- It's a great idea to use a blank journal or notebook along with this Eating Awareness Journal to continue writing and exploring based on the information and insights you uncover here.

SPECIAL REPORT

5 Ways Journaling Can STOP A BINGE

Do You Struggle to Avoid a Binge?

Are you Unable to Stop Once You Start?

Those of us who struggle with binge eating know that a binge can seem difficult to avoid and - once it starts - nearly impossible to stop. From the moment the idea takes root, even though we know we should resist that piece of cake and choose instead our peace of mind, a binge just seems inevitable.

Anything from sadness, fear or anger to tenderness, love or joy can become overwhelming – and we may not even notice what's happening until we're halfway through a box of chocolate chip cookies or we've taken a dive headfirst into a pint of praline ice cream.

This report will show you five ways journaling can **STOP YOUR NEXT BINGE.**

5 WAYS
JOURNALING CAN STOP A BINGE

DISTRACTION

Journaling gives you time and space to calm your mind. It helps by putting distance between you and your cravings.

Distraction can be enough to stop a binge.

AWARENESS

Ask yourself "what would nourish me in this moment?"

Awareness can be enough to stop a binge.

INSIGHT

Understanding why you eat to excess makes it possible to change your behavior.

Insight can be enough to stop a binge.

ACCOUNTABILITY

Accepting responsibility for your decisions and for your perspective allows you to make better, healthier choices.

Accountability can be enough to stop a binge.

SELF-CARE

If you listen to the messages from your true self, you can address the emotions that lead to overeating.

Self-care can be enough to stop a binge.

****

DISTRACTION

Get Ready to Shift Gears

If you feel yourself heading into or you're in the middle of a binge, you can interrupt the impulse by switching to something more constructive.

You could go for a walk, have a cup of tea, do some deep breathing, call a friend or take an exercise class. What I find works best is *writing in a journal*.

Journaling as Distraction

Journaling is an effective alternative to the over-consumption of chocolate. In the moment, it's not self-destructive. In the long-run, it's life-affirming.

When we journal, we give ourselves a break from feelings and emotions that are too intense. We remove ourselves from the source of anxiety. We give ourselves the distance we may need to collect our thoughts, take a step back and pay attention to what's really going on – how we feel physically and emotionally... and why.

How Does It Work?

As we focus on writing in our journal, time passes. Time may or may not heal all things... but if you can place enough time between your craving and the moment you head for the refrigerator or the bakery, that period of distraction can short-circuit your desire to binge. By the time you finish writing, your cravings may have less of a hold on you.

Journaling has been shown to reduce the anxiety that puts us at of risk over-eating. By expressing our thoughts and feelings in writing, getting them out of our head and onto paper, we can decrease their intensity and stop ourselves from barreling into over-eating. We can lessen both our stress and our cravings at the same time, with the stroke of a pen!

Start Now

Commit to writing in your journal the next time you feel a binge coming on, or find yourself in the middle of one. If it helps, tell yourself you can eat as soon as you finish writing, but give your journal a chance to change your mind.

Distraction may be enough to stop a binge.

Journaling Prompts

- What constructive activities could I choose when I feel anxious or stressed?

- What am I trying to avoid by eating/overeating?

- If I weren't eating, what would I be doing?

- What will I do as soon as I finish eating?

- Is there something I would rather be doing?

- Is there someone I would like to talk with right now? If so, what would I say?

- Is there something I'm putting off?

AWARENESS

Are You Eating on Autopilot?

Eating with the goal of satisfying cravings and ending anxiety moves us into auto-pilot. Once we're on the verge of, or in the middle of a binge, we're not thinking about *why* we want to eat, we just want to eat. Sure, there are times when we grab another cookie and wail, "why am I doing this?" It's not the same as letting go of that cookie and stopping to examine how we feel.

Does Examining Your Feelings Make You Anxious?

Maybe you're not so sure you want to know what you're feeling. After all, isn't that why we're eating in the first place -- to lessen the awareness that makes us so uncomfortable, to make sure we aren't dealing with too much, too soon or too intensely? We need that fried chicken, cupcake or treat to feel safe or sane.

Awareness at Your Own Pace

Journaling is a go-at-your-own pace exercise in self-awareness. When you pick up a pen and start journaling, you let the light in. You also control the amount that shines on you.

Out-of-control eating is a complex issue. Journaling can guide you to understanding while giving you a constructive way to deal with anxiety and stress.

Your journal will help you gain valuable insight into yourself and your relationship with food.

When we review what we've written in our journal, whether immediately or later, we often see why a trip to the vending machine or donut shop feels so tempting.

How Does It Work?

It's usually not just one idea that makes us anxious – it's a series of thoughts, feelings and beliefs. Our mind tries to process everything at once.

When we write, we break our thoughts into manageable pieces. It's less overwhelming that way. Less overwhelm means less of the anxiety that can lead to a binge or keep a binge going.

Start Now

Prepare by thinking of questions to ask yourself when you're in the grip of a binge. Start with the questions in this report. Write them into your journal, so that when you need them you can use them as prompts. Focus on self-awareness.

Awareness may be enough to stop a binge.

Journaling Prompts

- Am I hungry?

- What do I really want?

- Is there a food I feel I must have in this moment? Why is this food so important to me? Why now?

- How has the food I'm craving calmed me in the past? What is special about this food?

- What might be a healthier choice for me (for now or a later time)?

INSIGHT

Listen to Your Inner Voice

Your inner voice doesn't lie to you. It lets you know exactly what's there, beneath the surface. If you choose to listen, rather than judge yourself or your behavior, you can gain vital wisdom about yourself, your life and your relationship with food.

Your eating can help you identify areas of pain, stress, worry, fear and intense emotion, so you can begin to understand and compassionately heal them.

Make Connections

We can take an instance of out-of-control eating and, through writing about it, connect it to what may be less obvious. We can uncover our motivations, desires, fears and beliefs – the stories we tell ourselves and the way these stories play out in our lives. Insights don't have to be large to be helpful, they can be small observations about what leads us into the kitchen.

In the privacy of your journal, you can search for patterns, themes and cause-and-effect relationships; from deep, life-changing aha moments to simple "I never thought of that" discoveries.

Identify Your Habits

Habit chains are a series of events that are triggered, often by feelings or circumstances we don't notice. Once they start, we follow that familiar path to a bag of chips. At any point on our way to the bottom of that bag, we can break the chain – if we identify the links.

If your journal reveals that every time you pass a certain bakery, whether immediately or later that day, you end up eating an apple turnover, you can choose *not* to walk past that bakery.

Insight gives you the option to make a different choice.

How Does It Work?

Writing in your journal, even if you hold a fork in one hand and a pencil in the other, will reveal information and connections that allow you to make different decisions.

Awareness gives us the pieces. Insight puts them together.

The next time you feel pulled toward binge or are in the throes of binge behavior, set your intention to learn about yourself. Slow down, take a few breaths and tune into your mind and body, then send yourself a message of acceptance. Be open to compassionate understanding. Choose this moment to listen to your inner voice.

Insight may be enough to stop a binge.

Journaling Prompts

- If my binge eating was trying to say something, what would it tell me?

- If I trust that there is a good reason for my behavior, what is that reason? What need is being filled?

- What would nourish me right now? What kind of nourishment do I need? Will food provide this?

ACCOUNTABILITY

Look for Your Choice

Though we usually think of accountability as being "held accountable," by external forces such as bosses, parents, teachers or the legal system, in this case, we need to be accountable *to ourselves*.

In your journal, you can look for instances where you've turned a blind eye to your behavior with food. Nobody can make your choices for you or take them away from you.

You may not see where, in your current circumstance, your choice is hiding, but it's there. You have to look for it.

Choose Your Perspective

Your perspective defines your world: if you see your eating as bad or wrong, then (in your world), that's what it is. If you see yourself as helpless when faced with a dessert, that's what you are.

Imagine seeing things from a different angle. Imagine that the choice is yours – it is. You're the one grabbing that second slice.

Shift from thinking of your binge eating as an indictment of your worth to seeing it as vital information about yourself and the choices you make – information that could lead to a healthier, happier life.

You *can* choose your perspective. It's under your control.

Awaken New Possibilities

Accepting responsibility for the way you look at yourself and your life - and making it a point to seek out positive and healthy perspectives - will increase your self-esteem and empower you to change your circumstances. When you let go of a helpless mindset, and believe in your ability to bring about change, you awaken new possibilities.

How Does It Work?

Your journal is an opportunity to see the truth – your truth. Write about your current perspective when it comes to food and ask yourself how it helps you or hinders you. Then accept responsibility for holding onto or releasing that perspective. It's no small task, but it IS your choice. Hold yourself accountable.

Start Now

Pick one circumstance that leads to negative thoughts or feelings and see if you can adopt a more positive perspective. It might change the way you feel. It may even lessen the distress that threatens to send you careening into a binge.

Accountability may be enough to stop a binge.

Journaling Prompts

- Why am I choosing food at this moment? How does food address the current situation?

- Can I choose an activity other than eating?

- What is preventing me from making a different choice?

- Is it the food I really want?

- How will I feel after eating? What will be different? Is this the outcome I was seeking?

SELF-CARE

What Will Nourish You?

On the surface, binge eating is all about the food – food that feeds us without nourishing us. What if, when we're in the throes of a binge, instead of asking what we'll eat next, we ask "what would really nourish me right now?"

What Do You Really Need?

Through journaling, we can we can uncover the little lies we tell ourselves, the faulty connections we make and the effects of our current perspectives. By looking closely at ourselves, we can get a handle on what we really need and what we can do to take better care of ourselves.

Don't Miss the Lesson

Journaling is an immersion into self, which makes it the perfect place to explore and express emotions we might be eating to avoid.

Unless you show or share your journal, nobody else will see what you write. You don't need to be polite. Go ahead and complain, whine, criticize or say whatever you might not say in public.

If you think only a cupcake can make life bearable, write that down. If a cupcake is the best way to take care of yourself ... your journal will help you discover why.

How Does It Work?

When you write, you give yourself the time and space to listen to your inner voice. Instead of doing your best to forget those episodes of out-of-control eating, choose to look more closely at them and learn, so you can discover what you're expressing through food and choose a different behavior.

Your needs for self-care are always evolving. Your journal will keep you current with yourself and centered as changes occur... all while helping you evolve toward new and better choices. The more you learn about and express yourself, the less you need that binge.

Start Now

When you have a strong desire to overeat, think of it as a message from your true self. Listen without judgement and accept your truth. Banish blame and shame and replace them with compassion.

Self-care may be enough to stop a binge.

Journaling Prompts

- What is the kindest thing I could do for myself in this moment?

- What answers do I urgently need right now?

- What do I most need to express right now?

- How would I wish to be taken care of in this moment?

- How can I take care of myself in this moment?

****

MOTIVATIONS

What are the reasons you want to change your eating behavior? Write about your "why."

Whether our motivations are positive or negative, looking at them helps us understand ourselves. Developing insight into why we do what we do, gives us the power to change our thinking and our direction. Look with compassion at what motivates you.

Ask yourself if your reasons for wanting to change your relationship with food are positive or negative. If they feel more negative, do your best to restate them so they become an inspiration rather a source of fear or anxiety.

Studies show that focusing on what we want rather than what we don't want is effective in helping us achieve our goals, weight loss included.

Make this section one you'll return to again and again to remind you of the benefits of achieving your goals and taking control of your eating behavior. Use this section to reinforce your motivation.

\I encourage you to go to the back of this book where you'll find additional journaling pages. You might also want to get yourself a blank journal to use along with this one, so that you can more completely explore your insights and ideas. I love the wide variety of beautiful journals by Premise Content. Find a journal you love and keep writing!

A person often meets his destiny on the road he took to avoid it.

-Jean de La Fontaine

Why do I want to change my behavior?

How will I feel physically when I change my behavior?

How will I feel emotionally when I change my behavior?

How will I benefit from changing my behavior?

How will others benefit when I change my behavior?

What will be different when I change my behavior?

TOP FIVE MOTIVATIONS

1. _____

2. _____

3. _____

4. _____

5. _____

Let us not look back in anger, or forward in fear, but around in awareness.

-James Thurber

EATING AWARENESS

Words of Emotion

Abandoned	Edgy	Insulted	Sarcastic
Accommodating	Elated	Irritated	Satisfied
Afraid	Embarrassed	Isolated	Respected
Agitated	Empty	Interested	Rewarded
Alarmed	Energetic	Intimidated	Ridiculed
Alienated	Engaged	Jealous	Sad
Antagonistic	Enthusiastic	Joyful	Safe
Anxious	Excited	Judgmental	Scared
Apathetic	Fatigued	Jumpy	Secure
Apprehensive	Fearful	Lonely	Seething
Ashamed	Festive	Lost	Selfish
Awful	Flexible	Loved	Sensitive
Bad	Fragile	Loving	Shocked
Bitter	Free	Mad	Skeptical
Bold	Frightened	Needy	Startled
Bored	Frustrated	Neglected	Stressed
Bothered	Fulfilled	Numb	Supportive
Busy	Furious	Open	Suspicious
Competitive	Gleeful	Optimistic	Tactful
Concerned	Gloomy	Overwhelmed	Tenacious
Confident	Good	Panicky	Tender
Conflicted	Grateful	Passionate	Tense
Confused	Grieving	Patient	Terrified
Conspicuous	Grouchy	Peaceful	Testy
Courageous	Guilty	Perplexed	Threatened
Covetous	Happy	Petulant	Tired
Critical	Harassed	Playful	Tolerant
Defensive	Hesitant	Pleased	Touched
Depressed	Hopeful	Powerful	Tranquil
Despairing	Hopeless	Powerless	Triggered
Disappointed	Hostile	Prideful	Trusting
Disapproving	Humble	Provocative	Uneasy
Disgusted	Humiliated	Provoked	Unfair
Disillusioned	Hurt	Quarrelsome	Unnerved
Dismayed	Ignored	Reasonable	Victimized
Disrespected	Inadequate	Reckless	Virtuous
Distant	Indifferent	Rejected	Vulnerable
Distracted	Inferior	Relaxed	Weak
Distraught	Infuriated	Remorseful	Withdrawn
Distressed	Insecure	Repugnant	Worried
Eager	Insignificant	Restless	Worthless
Ecstatic	Inspired	Resentful	Worthy

Week One

Date: _____

Time	Food and Drink	How I Feel		
		Before Eating	During	After Eating

Date: _____

Time	Food and Drink	How I Feel		
		Before Eating	During	After Eating

Date: _____

Time	Food and Drink	How I Feel		
		Before Eating	During	After Eating

Date: _____

Time	Food and Drink	How I Feel		
		Before Eating	During	After Eating

38

Date: _____

Time	Food and Drink	How I Feel		
		Before Eating	During	After Eating

Date: _____

Time	Food and Drink	How I Feel		
		Before Eating	During	After Eating

42

Date: _____

Time	Food and Drink	How I Feel		
		Before Eating	During	After Eating

Week One INSIGHTS

Overall, this week was:

_____

_____

_____

How I felt this week:

What insights and connections have I noticed this week?

_____
_____
_____
_____
_____
_____
_____
_____
_____

What patterns have I noticed this week?

_____
_____
_____
_____
_____
_____
_____
_____
_____

Suggestions for next week?

_____
_____
_____
_____
_____
_____
_____
_____
_____
_____
_____

Focus for next week:

1.
_____

2.
_____

3.
_____

Week Two

Date: _____

Time	Food and Drink	How I Feel		
		Before Eating	During	After Eating

Date: _____

Time	Food and Drink	How I Feel		
		Before Eating	During	After Eating

54

Date: _____

Time	Food and Drink	How I Feel		
		Before Eating	During	After Eating

Date: _____

Time	Food and Drink	How I Feel		
		Before Eating	During	After Eating

58

Date: _____

Time	Food and Drink	How I Feel		
		Before Eating	During	After Eating

Date: _____

Time	Food and Drink	How I Feel		
		Before Eating	During	After Eating

Date: _____

Time	Food and Drink	How I Feel		
		Before Eating	During	After Eating

64

Week Two INSIGHTS

Overall, this week was:

_____

_____

_____

How I felt this week:

What insights and connections have I noticed this week?

_____
_____
_____
_____
_____
_____
_____
_____

What patterns have I noticed this week?

_____
_____
_____
_____
_____
_____
_____
_____

Suggestions for next week?

_____
_____
_____
_____
_____
_____
_____
_____
_____
_____

Focus for next week:

1.
_____

2.
_____

3.
_____

Week Three

Date: _____

Time	Food and Drink	How I Feel		
		Before Eating	During	After Eating

Date: _____

Time	Food and Drink	How I Feel		
		Before Eating	During	After Eating

74

Date: _____

Time	Food and Drink	How I Feel		
		Before Eating	During	After Eating

76

Date: _____

Time	Food and Drink	How I Feel		
		Before Eating	During	After Eating

Date: _____

Time	Food and Drink	How I Feel		
		Before Eating	During	After Eating

Date: _____

Time	Food and Drink	How I Feel		
		Before Eating	During	After Eating

Date: _____

Time	Food and Drink	How I Feel		
		Before Eating	During	After Eating

Week Three INSIGHTS

Overall, this week was:

_____

_____

_____

How I felt this week:

What insights and connections have I noticed this week?

_____
_____
_____
_____
_____
_____
_____
_____

What patterns have I noticed this week?

_____
_____
_____
_____
_____
_____
_____
_____

Suggestions for next week?

_____

_____

_____

_____

_____

_____

_____

_____

_____

_____

_____

Focus for next week:

1.
_____

2.
_____

3.
_____

Week Four

Date: _____

Time	Food and Drink	How I Feel		
		Before Eating	During	After Eating

Date: _____

Time	Food and Drink	How I Feel		
		Before Eating	During	After Eating

Date: _____

Time	Food and Drink	How I Feel		
		Before Eating	During	After Eating

96

Date: _____

Time	Food and Drink	How I Feel		
		Before Eating	During	After Eating

Date: _____

Time	Food and Drink	How I Feel		
		Before Eating	During	After Eating

Date: _____

Time	Food and Drink	How I Feel		
		Before Eating	During	After Eating

Date: _____

Time	Food and Drink	How I Feel		
		Before Eating	During	After Eating

Week Four INSIGHTS

Overall, this week was:

_____

_____

_____

How I felt this week:

What insights and connections have I noticed this week?

_____
_____
_____
_____
_____
_____
_____
_____

What patterns have I noticed this week?

_____
_____
_____
_____
_____
_____
_____
_____

Suggestions for next week?

_____

_____

_____

_____

_____

_____

_____

_____

_____

_____

Focus for next week:

1.
_____

2.
_____

3.
_____

JOURNAL PAGES

ABOUT DAVINA

Davina Chessid is an author and life coach in New York City. Her book **Food Crazy Mind** has been an Amazon bestseller in multiple categories.

Davina's struggle with out-of-control eating has helped her understand, connect and work effectively with clients facing a similar challenge.

If you suffer from compulsive eating, over-eating, binge-eating or emotional eating – and the reduced quality of life that accompanies these – you're not alone.

Find the book Food Crazy Mind on Amazon.com, along with a variety of Food Crazy Mind journals.

Visit Davina at: foodcrazymind.com.

If you love to journal, look for a wide selection of blank and guided journals by Premise Content at premisecontent.com or visit Premise Content on Amazon.com.

Other Food Crazy Mind Journals:

Daily Food Journal

Eating Awareness for Binge Eaters

Food & Feelings Journal

Have you read Food Crazy Mind?

Find it on Amazon.com.

Visit my page on Amazon at:

amazon.com/author/davinachessid

or

visit me at my website: www.foodcrazymind.com.

Made in the USA
Columbia, SC
29 May 2020